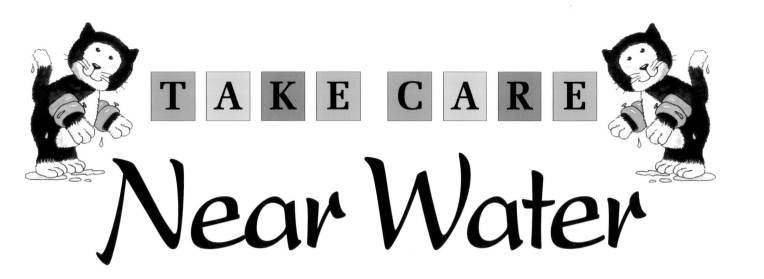

TAKE CARE

Near Water

Carole Wale

RoSPA

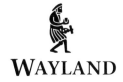

WAYLAND

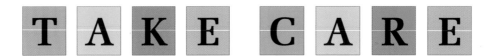

TAKE CARE

At Home   On Your Own
Near Water   On the Road

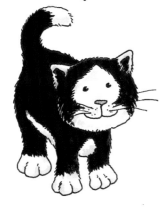

Editors: Katie Orchard and Sarah Doughty
Designer: Jean Wheeler
Artist: Lynne Farmer
Production controller: Carol Titchener

First published in 1996 by Wayland Publishers Ltd
61 Western Road, Hove,
East Sussex BN3 1JD

British Library Cataloguing in Publication Data
Wale, Carole
Take care near water
1. Aquatic sports – Safety measures – Juvenile literature
2. Drowning – Prevention – Juvenile literature
3. Safety measures – Juvenile literature
I. Title
363.1'23'083

ISBN 0 7502 1786 3

Typeset by Jean Wheeler, in England
Printed and bound in England by B.P.C. Paulton Books

Picture credits: All photographs by Angus Blackburn except J Allan Cash 23 (top);
Piers Cavendish/Impact cover, 7, 14, 15 (bottom), 16, 17 (top), 18 (bottom), 19, 22, 24, 25;
and Bruce Stephens/Impact 4, 8, 9, 10, 11 (both), 12, 13, 20 (both), 21.

Contents

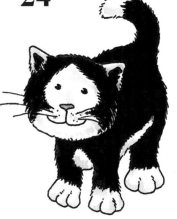

The words that appear in **bold** are explained
in the picture glossary on page 30.

Water in the Home

Water is important. We need water to live and we use it every day of our lives.

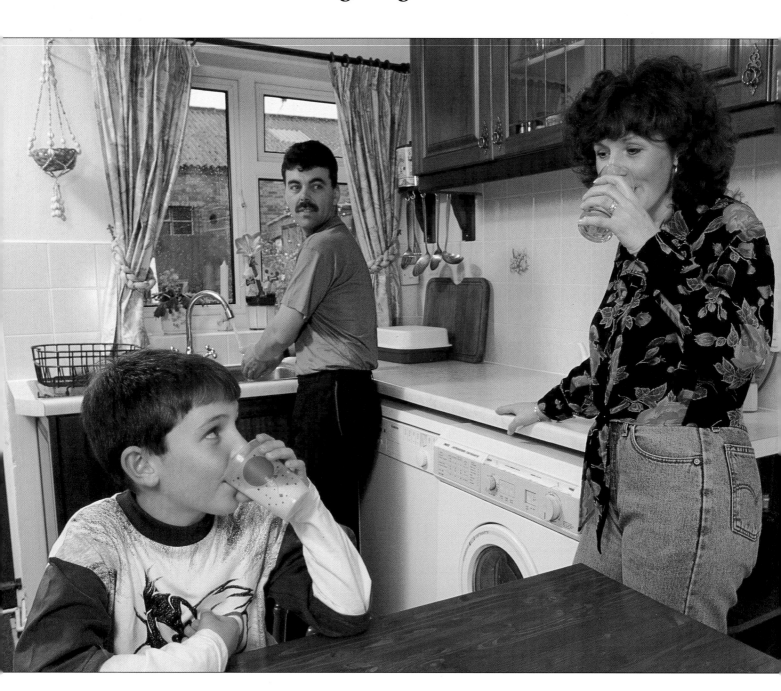

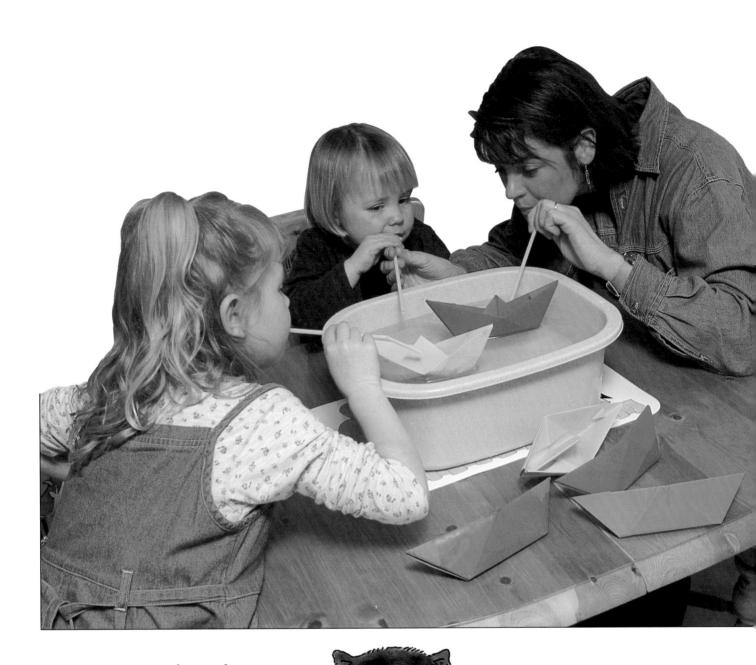

We can also have
fun and play with
water if we take
care.

Always have
an adult with
you when you
are near water.

In the Garden

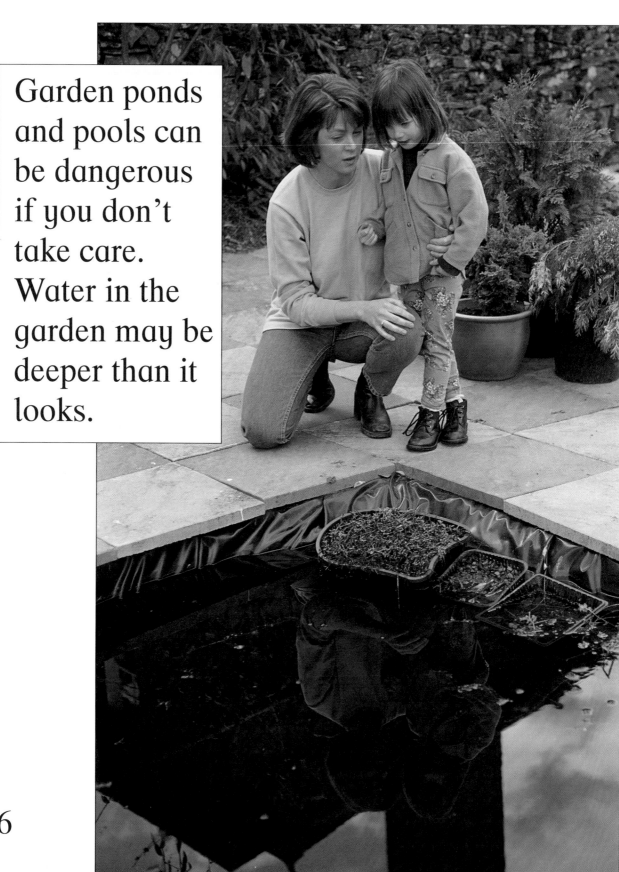

Garden ponds and pools can be dangerous if you don't take care. Water in the garden may be deeper than it looks.

If you have a **paddling pool**, ask an adult to empty it as soon as you have finished using it.

Be very careful near water butts or water barrels. When it rains they can get very full.

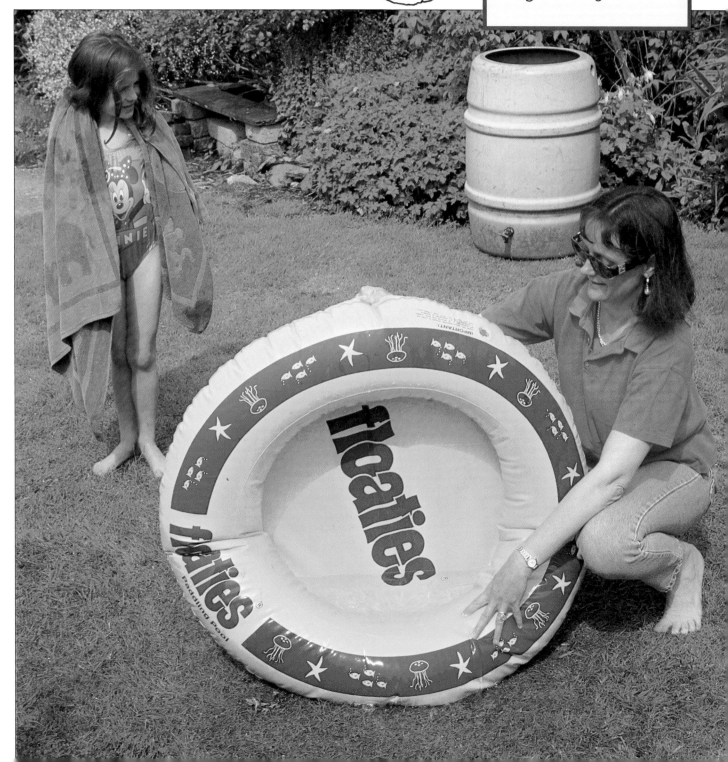

Learning to Swim

Learning to swim is good for you. It can also be fun. Swimming helps to keep you strong and healthy.

At the pool, a swimming **instructor** can help you learn to swim.

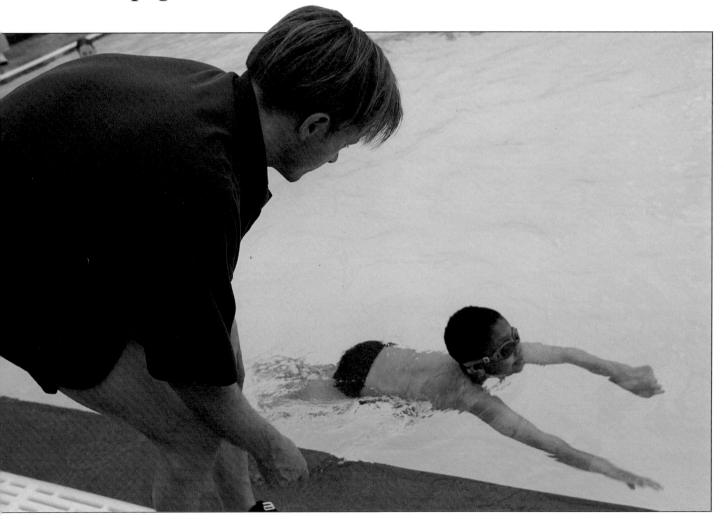

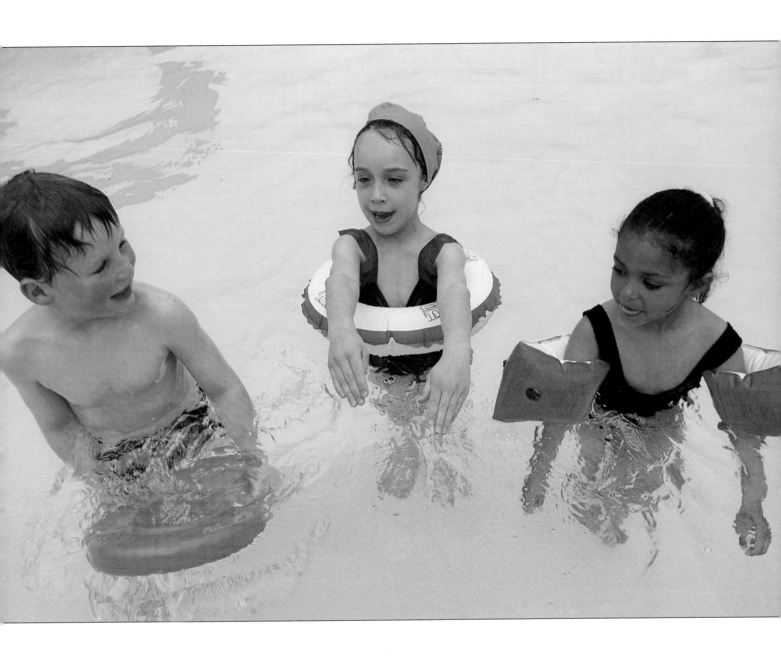

You can use **inflatable** arm bands, rubber rings and **floats** to help you learn to swim.

Some swimming baths have a special pool where children can learn to swim. The pool is warm, clean and **supervised**.

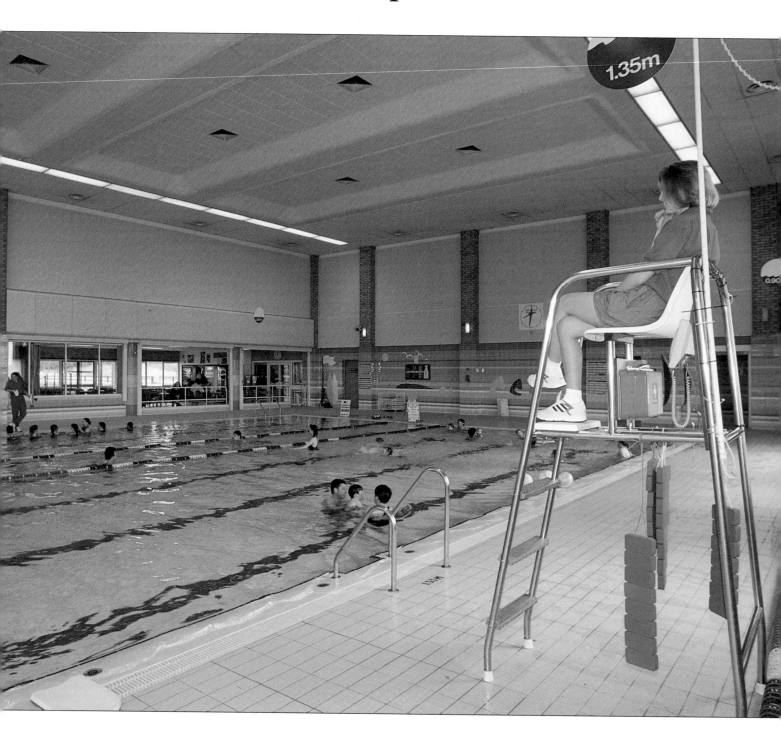

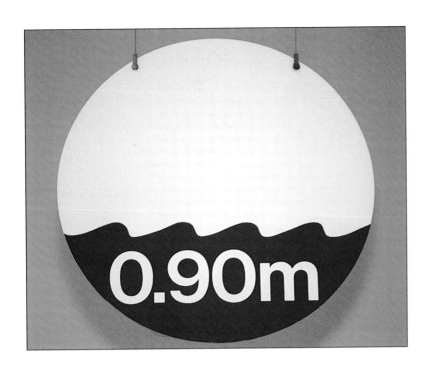

Always stay
in the shallow end
until you can swim
properly. Make sure
your feet can
touch the floor.

Along the pool you will find notices to tell you how deep the water is.

There will be a **shallow** end and a deep end.

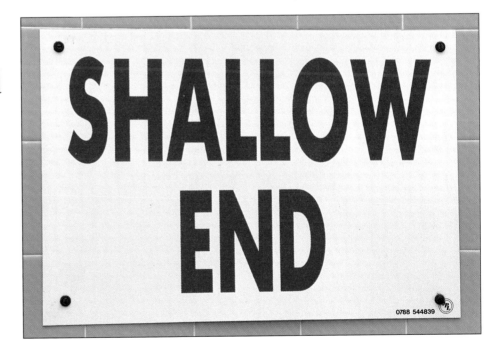

SHALLOW END

0788 544839

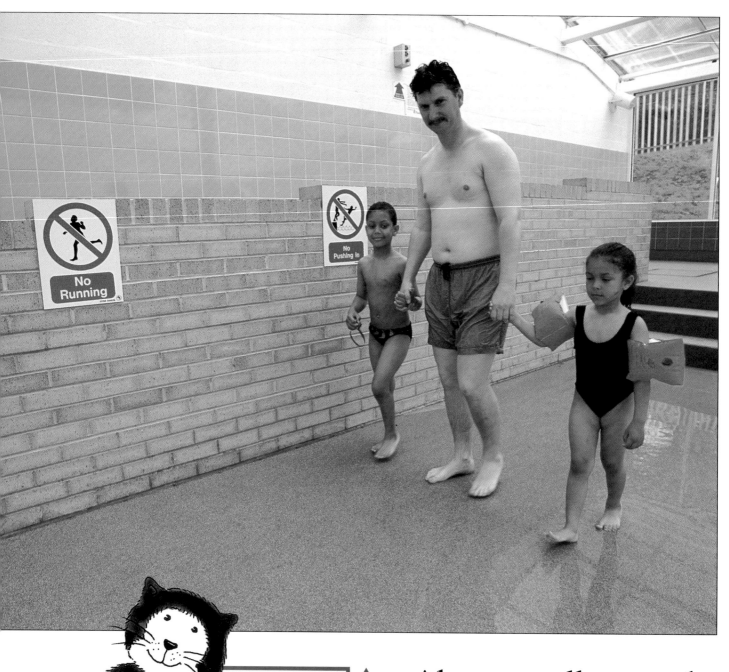

Always walk around the swimming pool as the tiles get wet and slippery. You might fall if you run.

Make sure you look before getting into the water. There may be someone already in the water.

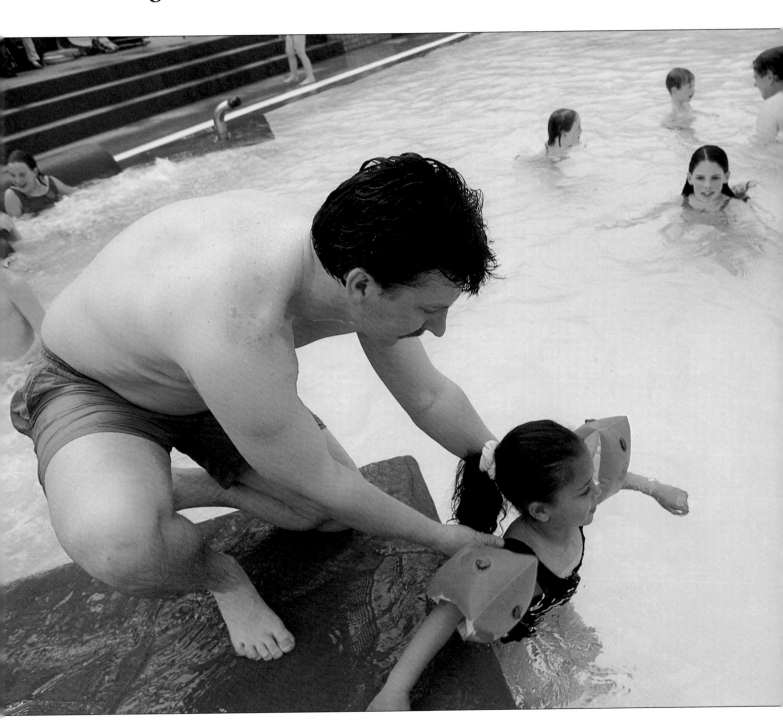

Parks and Playgrounds

Ponds and pools in parks and near playgrounds are not like indoor swimming pools.

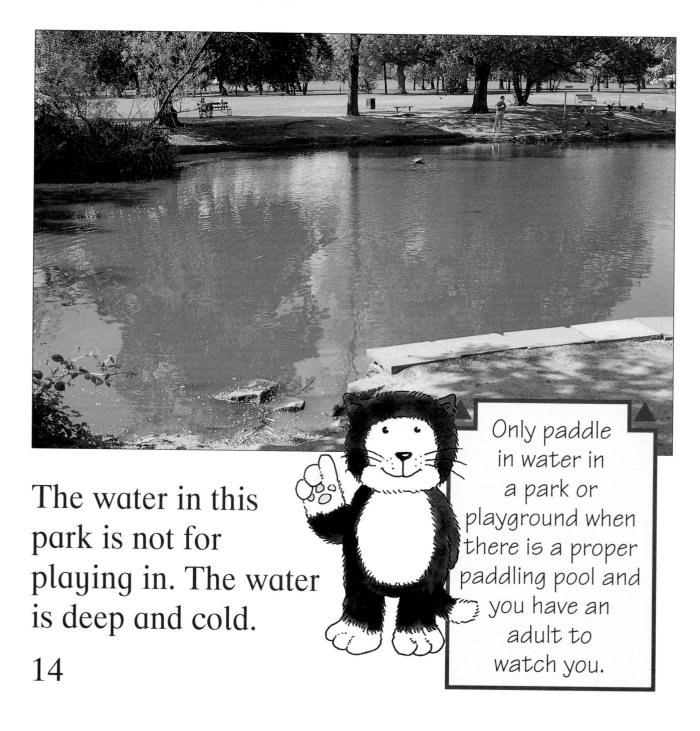

The water in this park is not for playing in. The water is deep and cold.

Only paddle in water in a park or playground when there is a proper paddling pool and you have an adult to watch you.

Water flows
quickly in a park
waterfall. You can
watch it, but don't
go too close.

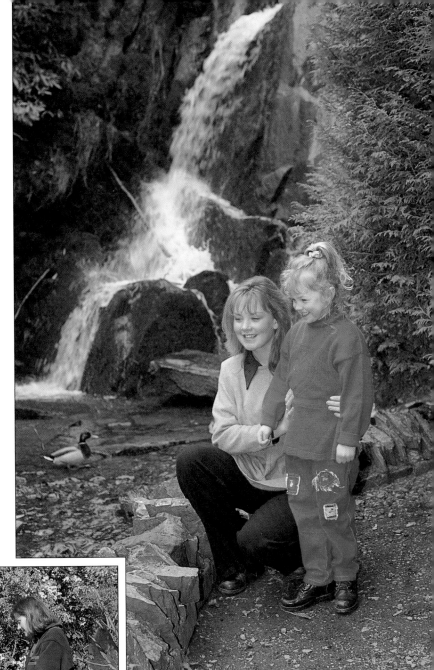

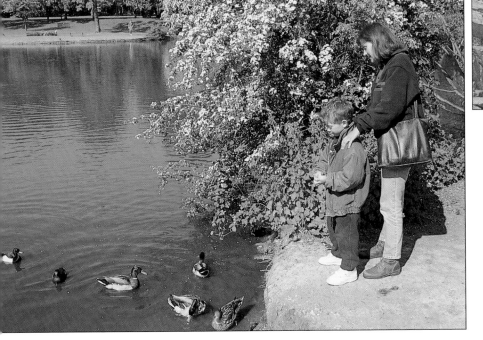

You can feed
the ducks on
the pond but
take care.

Farms and the Countryside

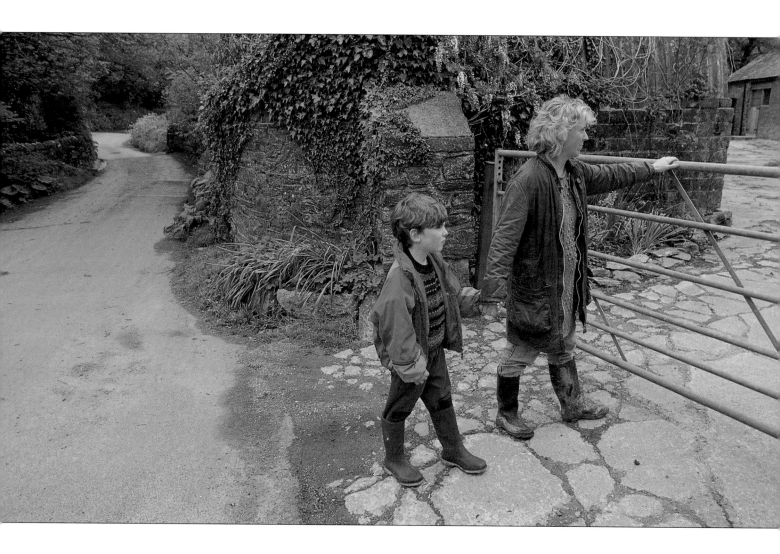

This is the entrance to a farm.

There are many water dangers on farmland and in the countryside.

16

When the land **floods**, there can be puddles. The water is often cold and very dirty. This field is wet and muddy.

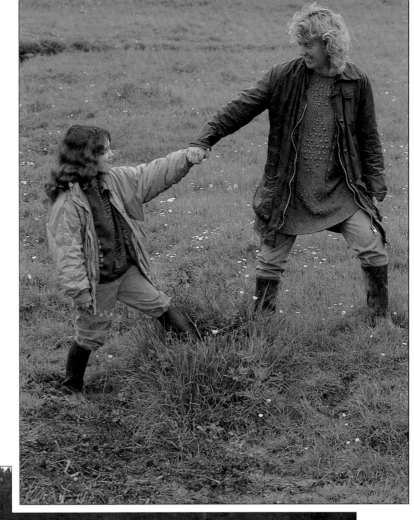

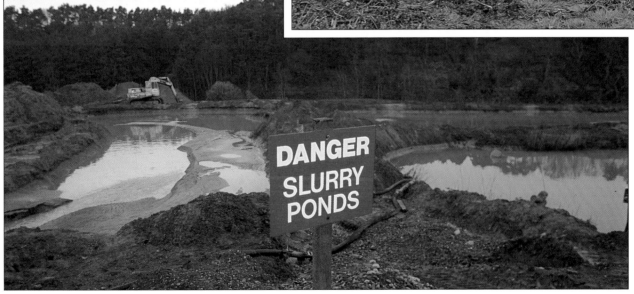

Keep away from water tanks, **cattle troughs** and **slurry ponds**, as you may fall in.

Streams and Rivers

Be careful near rivers and streams as there are often strong **currents** beneath the surface.

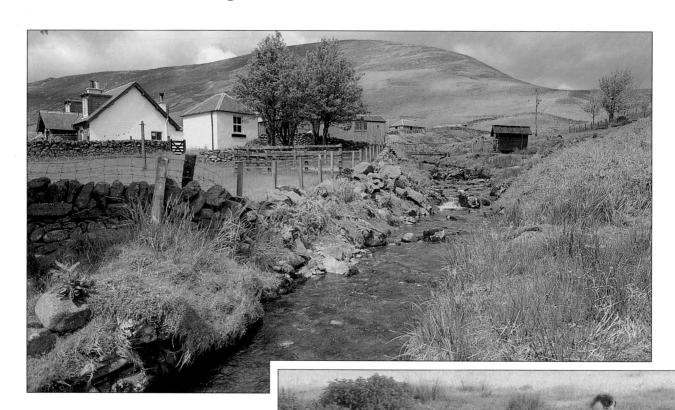

This stream is fast-flowing. The floor is rocky and it may be slippery at the edges.

This river is deep and cold, even on a fine, sunny day.

Never try and swim in a river even if you can swim well in an indoor pool.

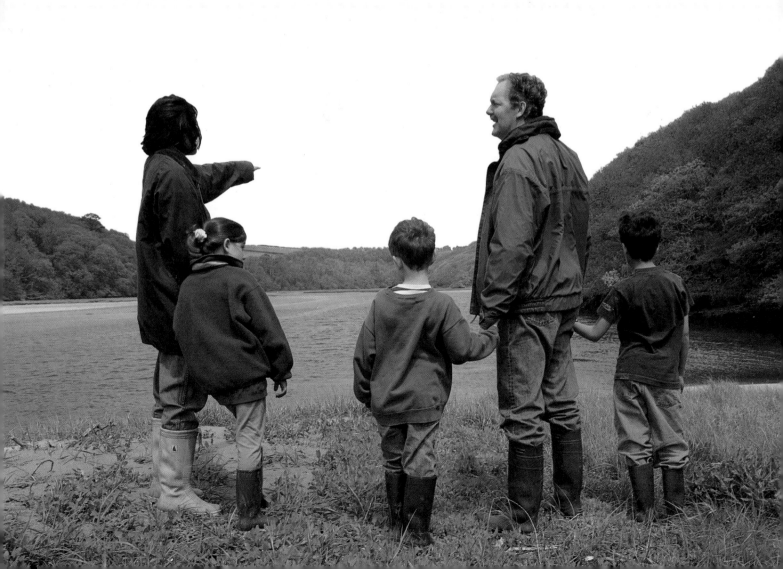

Canals

A canal is a
waterway.
The water in
a canal can be
very deep.

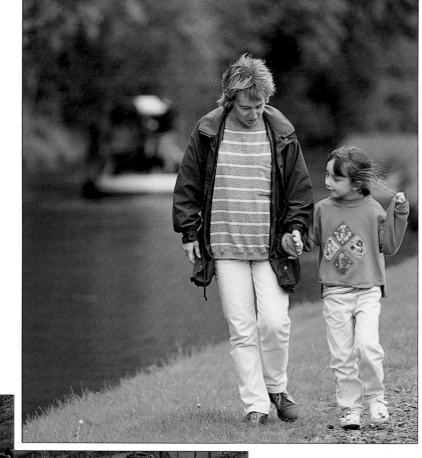

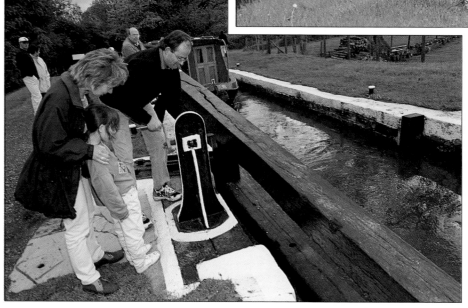

These are lock gates on a canal.
Locks are dangerous if you are not
careful. The sides are steep and
water flows into the lock very fast.

Canals and rivers have large boats
on them, like this narrowboat.
Never play near boats.

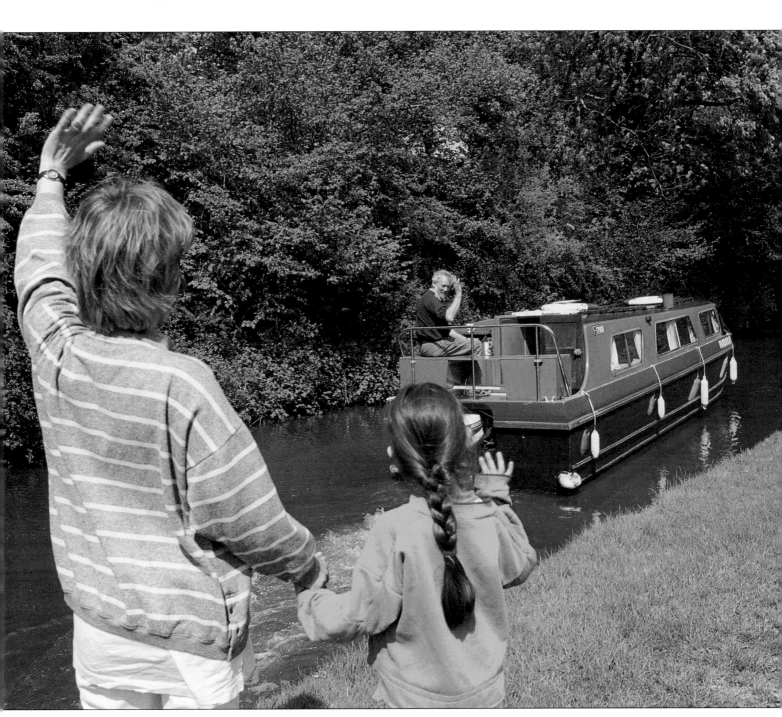

Reservoirs and Lakes

Reservoirs are used for storing water.

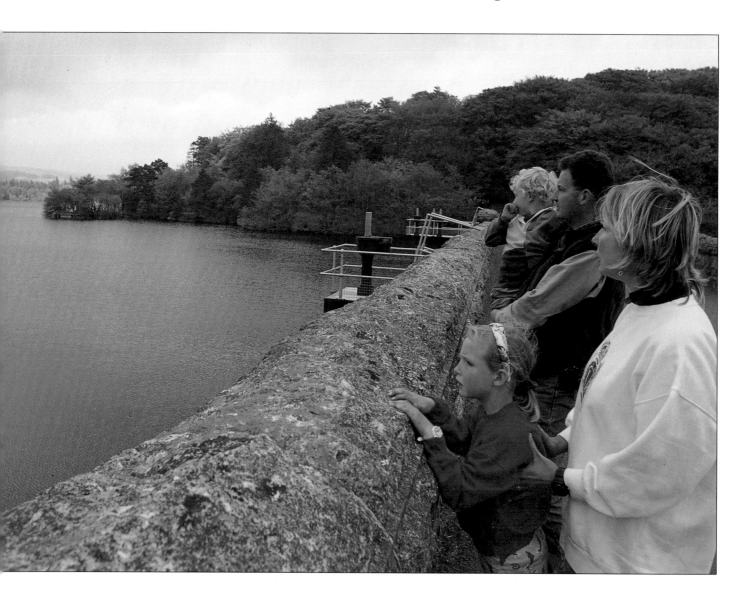

Reservoirs and lakes are very deep and the water is always cold, even when the weather is hot on a summer's day.

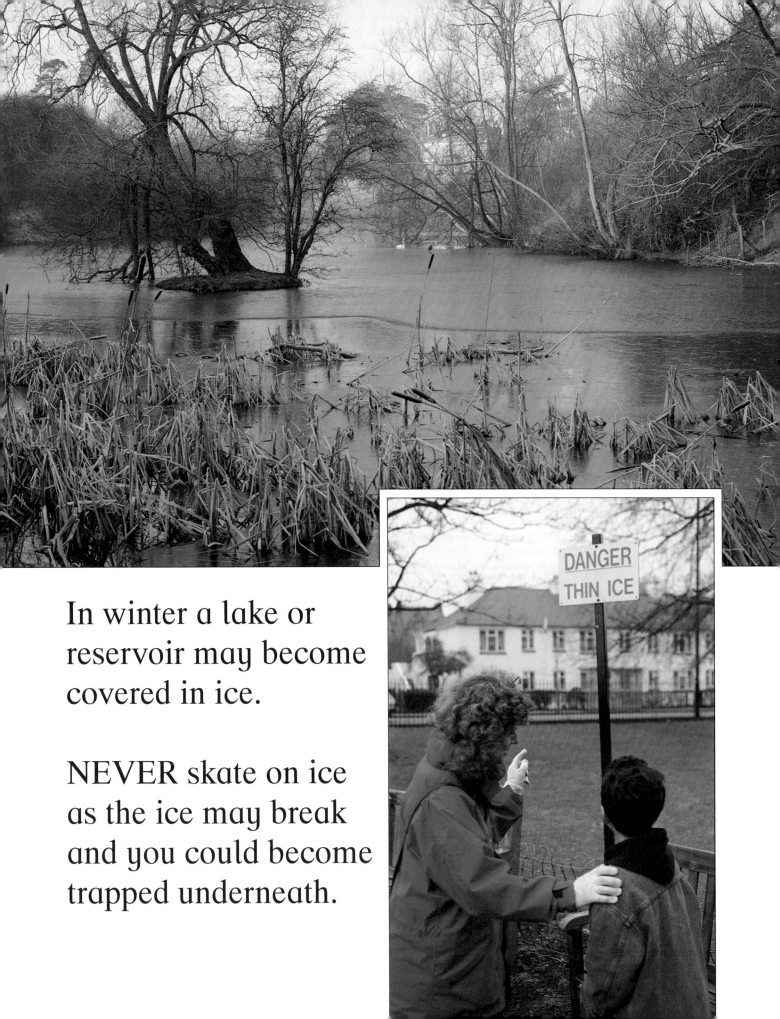

In winter a lake or reservoir may become covered in ice.

NEVER skate on ice as the ice may break and you could become trapped underneath.

At the Seaside

The sea has **tides** and **currents** which can change suddenly and it is very cold. Never use inflatables on the sea as you could drift into deep water.

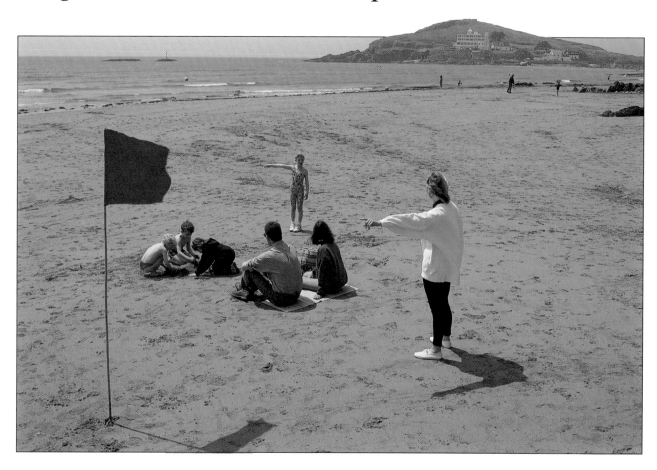

If you see a red flag flying on the beach, do not go into the water. The red flag means DANGER.

Watch out for sharp objects, pebbles
and shells on the beach and in the sea.
Take care that you don't cut your feet.

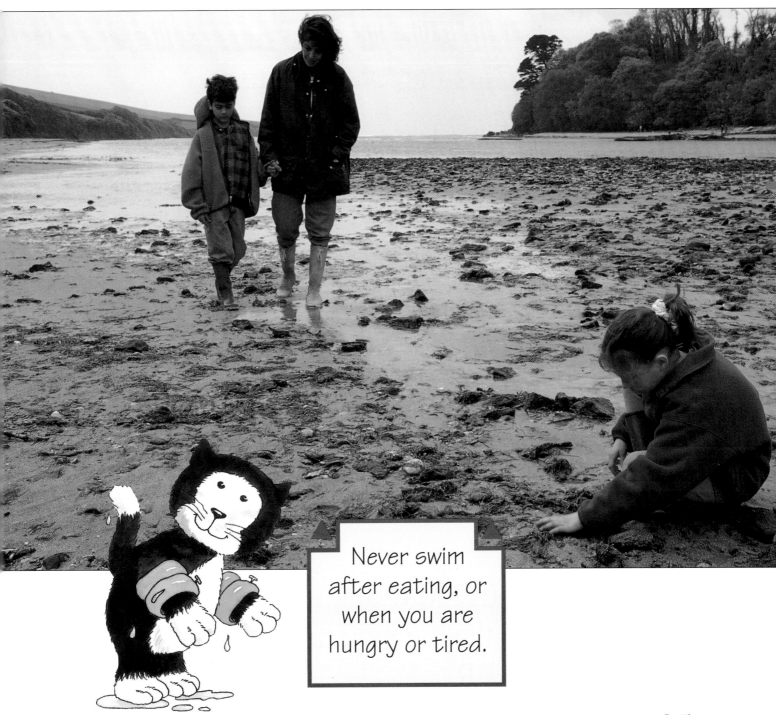

Never swim
after eating, or
when you are
hungry or tired.

In Boats

Always wear a **life-jacket** when you get into a boat, even if you can swim.

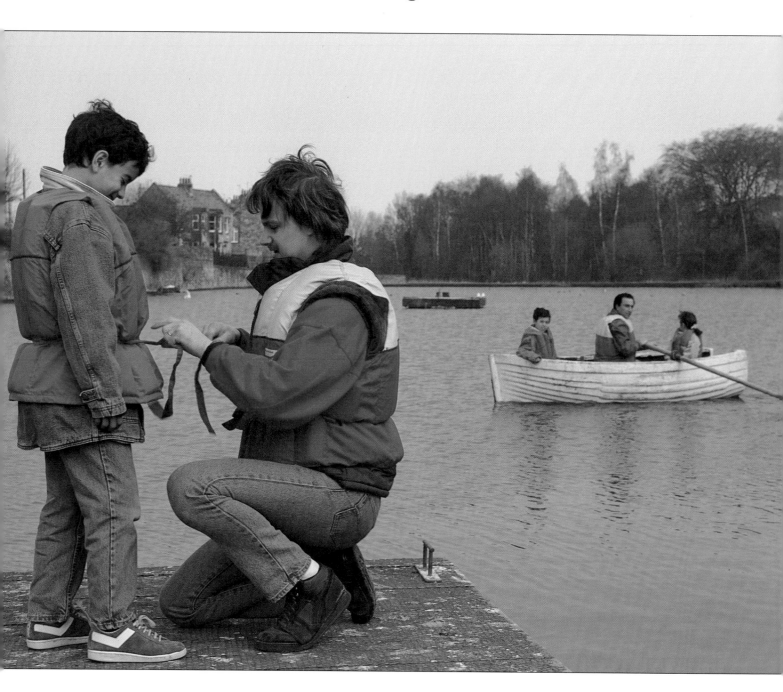

Always sit down in the boat.
It is safer for you.

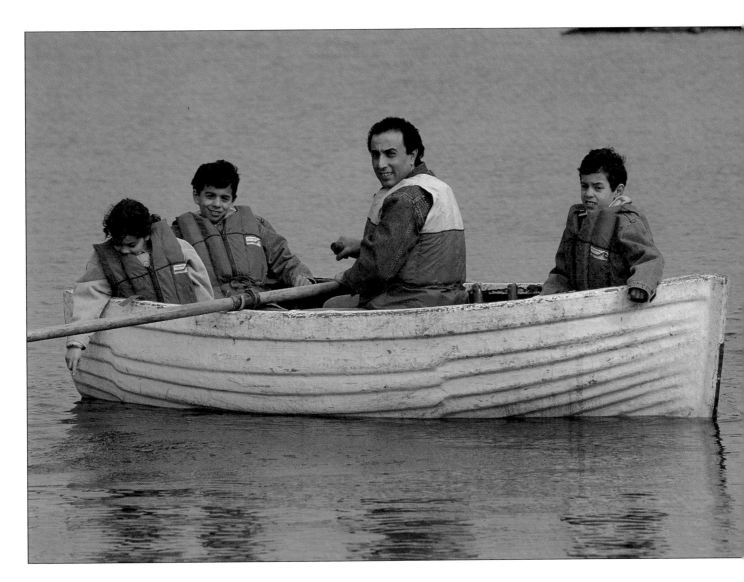

When you look over the sides of the boat,
never lean out too far over the water.

Be Safe at the Pool

Who is behaving safely at the swimming pool? Who is being unsafe?

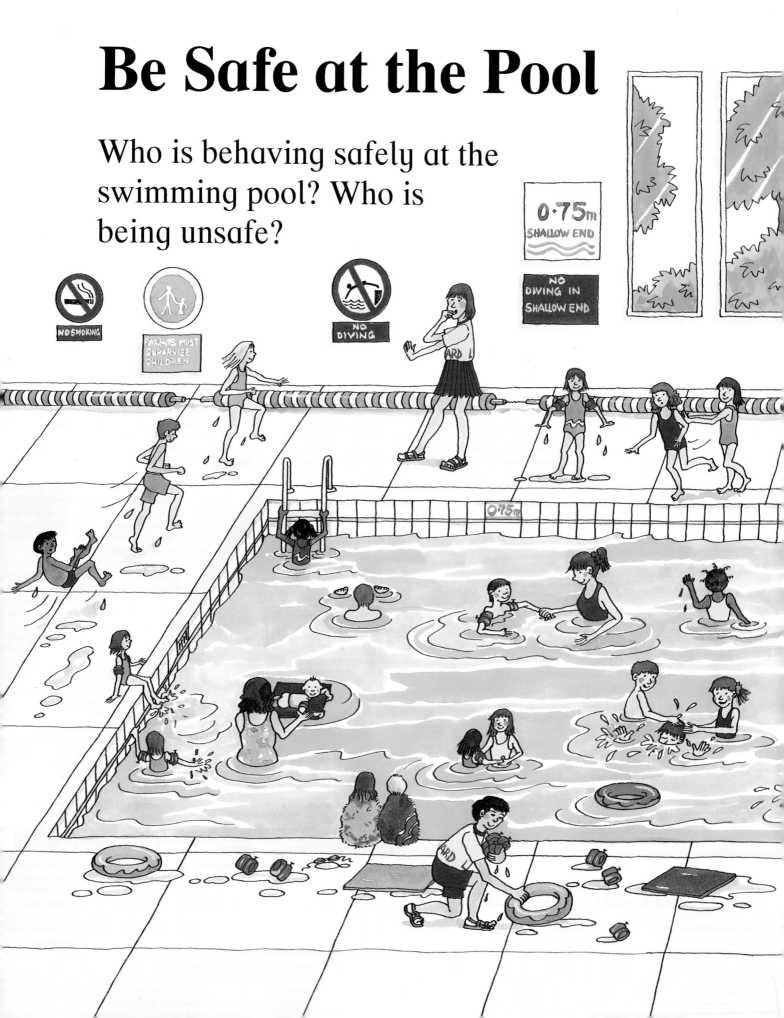

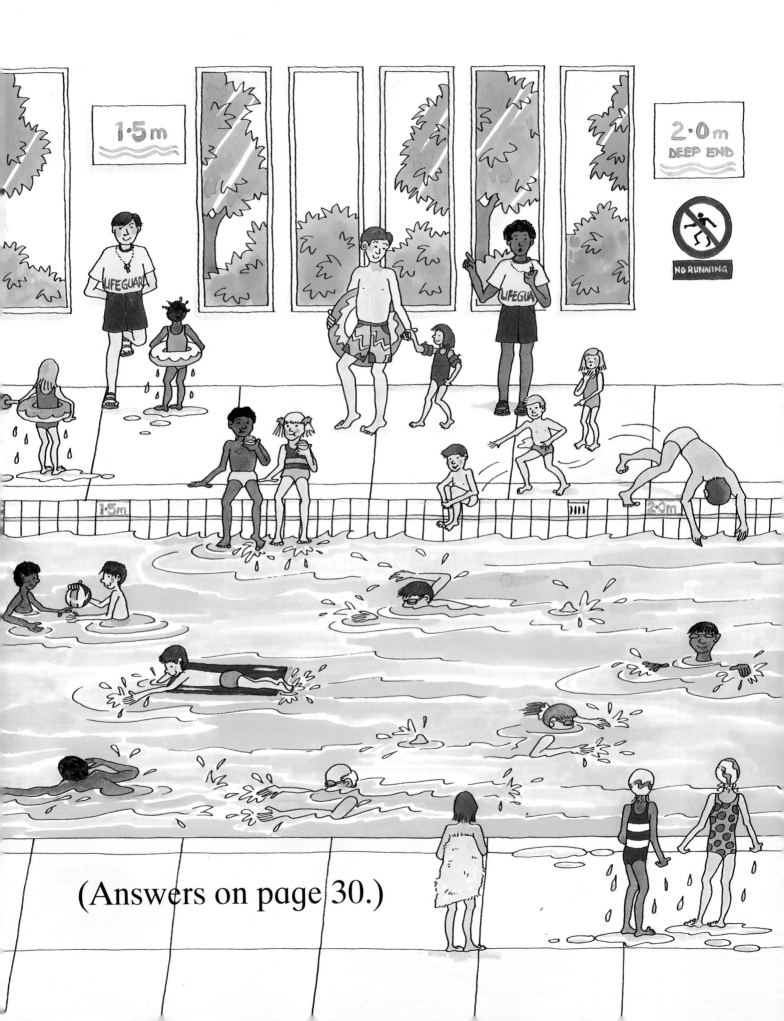

(Answers on page 30.)

Picture Glossary

 canals Stretches of deep water with locks. Large boats travel on them.

 cattle troughs Containers on farms used for feeding animals.

 current The strong movement of the water in one direction.

 floats Small cork boards which you can hold when you learn to swim. They float in water.

 flood When rivers, streams and other types of water overflow on to the land.

 inflatable When something can be filled with air to help you float in water.

 instructor Someone who can tell you how to do something safely.

 life-jacket An inflatable, brightly coloured jacket worn by people on boats.

 paddling pool An inflatable pool used in the garden. It is too shallow for swimming in.

 shallow Not very deep.

 slurry ponds Deep wells on farms that contain thin, sloppy mud.

 supervised Where someone is watching you to keep you safe.

 tides The way the sea rises and falls. Tides can be very powerful.

 water tanks Large, metal containers which store water.

Answers to pages 28-9: Unsafe people include the child running around the slippery edge of the pool; the children jumping or diving in the pool near other swimmers, the children ducking another child underwater, the child pushing another into the pool, the children eating on the edge of the pool. Safe people include: the child wearing water wings with a supervising adult, the mother and baby in the shallow end of the pool, children and adults swimming sensibly, the child using the steps to get in and out of the pool, the child holding the hand of an adult to walk around the edge of the pool.

Books to Read

I Can Swim by Sheila Fraser and Lisa Kopper (Aladdin Books, 1991)

Look Out by Water by Helena Ramsay (Evans Brothers Ltd, 1994)

The Be Water Wise Book (RoSPA Publications, 1990)

Watch Out! Near Water by Anne Smith (Wayland, 1991)

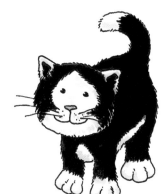

Notes for Parents and Teachers

Most children love water. Water play and water sport can be fun but are also dangerous. Young children can drown in just a few centimetres of water. The ability to swim does not solve the problem. Around three-quarters of those who drown can swim.

Children should be taught to swim at a young age. They need to develop water confidence, but they also need to develop a healthy respect for water and to understand its many dangers. It is never too early to teach children the simple rules of water safety.

Children should be taught to swim by professional instructors in well supervised pools where safety is a prime consideration. Remind children that swimming in a warm, supervised indoor pool is not the same as swimming in the sea or outdoors.

Always supervise children when they are near water. Children should not be allowed on their own near ponds, lakes, canals or rivers.

The seaside also has many hazards for children.

Teach them about the unique nature of the sea, its power, the tides and the waves. Children should never take inflatable beds or toys into the sea as they could easily drift into deep waters. Make sure that they know about other hazards such as slippery rocks and pebbles in the water and on the beach.

Make sure that children know what to do when in boats, that they should always wear life-jackets and stay close to an adult. Teach children to recognize and understand the meanings of safety signs and warning notices and make sure that they obey them.

Whenever you are near water take the opportunity to discuss water safety. Make sure that children know the dangers, recognize the type of water and know how to behave accordingly. Water on farms and in the countryside needs special attention as children may not understand the hazards.

For further information about water safety, contact: RoSPA, Edgbaston Park, 353 Bristol Road, Birmingham, B5 75T.

Index

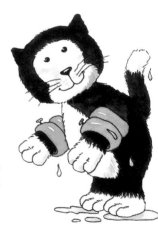